The Bottom Line

Getting a Grip on Your Practice's Finances

Ben Bradley

The Bottom Line
Getting a Grip on Your Practice's Finances
Printed by:
90-Minute Books
302 Martinique Drive
Winter Haven, FL 33884
www.90minutebooks.com

Published in the United States of America

Book ID: 160426-00406

ISBN-13: 978-1945733031
ISBN-10: 1945733039

For more information on 90-Minute Books including finding out how you can
publish your own lead generating book, visit www.90minutebooks.com or call
(863) 318-0464

Here's What's Inside…

The Bottom Line!

Congratulations, you have graduated from Dental and/or Medical school, you are in private practice and find yourself running a small business. You may now be asking yourself "When did I become an entrepreneur? I am an Oral Surgeon; I didn't go to school to run a business". You are not alone. Many surgeons even after years of school are never taught how to run a business. They're given the keys to a 7-figure business, but they don't always know exactly what to do with it.

Doctors dedicate their lives to making a difference in people's lives. Yet if you are around the industry long enough, you hear many stories about doctors who need to work well into their 70s in order to keep paying the bills. This could be because of the finite window of time surgeons have to actually make money after they are done with their training. After school they have to pay down their student debt (current cost of dental school is close to $90,000 per year) the debt they took on (or income lost) to buy into a practice, pay down the mortgage on office space and their home, put their children through college, and save for retirement; this is no small undertaking.

It's been very gratifying to be able to help my clients, surgeons like you, understand their bottom line and how they got there.

When you own the business, every dollar that comes into the business matters and when it goes to the wrong "bucket", or if there is overspending on supplies, personnel, equipment, etc. that comes out of your pocket, your family's pocket, and it adversely affects your personal finances in addition to your professional financial health it may mean you will have no choice other than to worker longer than you planned.

What I've found in working with my clients is that they need a translator or intermediary between the CPA (certified public accountant) and the doctor; a quarterback if you will. I work with my clients to translate everything that the CPA is saying and present all these complex financial statements in a way that my clients are able to quickly digest, understand and then use as a launching pad to be able to make sound business decisions.

There is often a light bulb moment when all of sudden the client will understand what all these numbers mean simply because it was presented to them in a new way. Everyone processes information differently and knowing how you learn or understand material is the first step in understanding your finances. You are paying your CPA good money to be a trusted advisor for you, and they are giving you invaluable information about your business. Understanding the information they are providing will get you the most out of that relationship and this is where I can help.

If you understand the five keys that I summarize in this book, you will be able to get a grip on your practice finances.

You will have a better understanding not only of where the money is going within your business, but, also how to plan for seasonal changes in cash flow.

I will show you the benefit of having goals. If you don't have goals and benchmarks then what are you really comparing yourself to? With these goals, you can then create a plan which you and your team can follow through on. You will see results allowing you to understand how your financial performance compares to other practices and your own practice historically.

I hope this book inspires you to truly understand where every dollar goes in your business, and educates you about what you need to do to be in control of your practice's finances.

Enjoy the book!

To Your Success!

Ben Bradley

Why Don't More Oral Surgeons Have Confidence and Understanding About Their Practice Financing?

Although oral surgeons spend years and years training to become surgeons, many are never taught how to evaluate financial reports. For them to do so would be like asking an accountant to evaluate a radiograph. Like many other small-business owners, doctors rely on experts in fields in which they're not well-versed. This may mean outsourcing tasks, such as bookkeeping or medical billing. It is okay to do this. You are not alone. For many practices, outsourcing is a great option because it allows business owners to focus on what they do best - surgery.

Once you, as an owner, have outsourced the financial analysis portion of running your business, and the CPA provides you with your financial reports throughout the year, it's extremely important that you ask questions to fully understand these reports. Often, a business owner becomes embarrassed because although they're running a successful business, have advanced degrees, and are extremely bright individuals, they don't always understand what all of their reports mean. Trust me you are not alone. The good news is that gaining an understanding of this is easier than many think. You just need to have a good grasp of the information in the form in which it is presented. You need to ask more questions, just like a patient would ask you questions about a condition or a procedure until they understand. Business owners need to do the same thing when their experts and advisors give them information.

They need to take the information given to them with the understanding that they're speaking with knowledgeable people in their fields.

Oftentimes, a surgeon doesn't fully grasp their practice finances because they've been so busy trying to grow their practice they don't often have the opportunity or bandwidth to look at the other side of their business, the numbers. Frankly, understanding finances is much easier than what a surgeon does on a day-to-day basis. There's a reason that they have dental school, medical school, and residency all after obtaining a bachelor's degree. It doesn't take that level of education to understand the finances of a small business.

Lack of knowledge about your practice's financials could prove to be detrimental to your financial health, both personally and professionally. Not understanding your financials is like trying to place an implant without a CBCT or X-ray. The sentiment becomes, "Well, that's close enough," rather than, "Yes, this is correct. This makes sense, and I agree with it."

Every day during surgery a surgeon has to know so much about the biology, chemistry, anatomy, and more, but they have never really been taught how to run a business. They spend so much time working on the clinical aspect of things that the business aspects of being a successful business owner often get left behind. Unless they have a business degree, which would require them to do even more schooling before enrolling in medical or dental school, they really don't have a lot of exposure to the business side.

Typically, a CPA is the right person to advise you on your finances. You should have a good working relationship with your accountant; your personalities should be a good match. A CPA is board certified; the fact that they are competent comes with obtaining the certification. They will be able to fulfill virtually all of your needs in the financial area of your business. So it becomes a matter of whether their personality is a good fit and whether or not they have experience in your industry. Not having experience in your industry does not preclude them from being a good fit for you, but, sometimes having a CPA with other clients in your industry only helps them be more effective. You want a CPA that will be a cultural, philosophical, and personality fit (down to communication). They are a business advisor for you and you want to be able to reach them when you have questions. At that point, it's really a matter of fine-tuning the information they provide.

Why Confidence and Understanding Leads to a Better Bottom Line

Having an understanding of your practice financing, really allows you to make more educated business decisions. You will be a better business owner. You will be able to say, "Things feel a little bit tight; I should have more cash," or, "I'm thinking about hiring another surgical assistant. Do I have the money for that?"

Once you have an understanding of your practice's finances, you will be able to figure out where you are overspending (or not generating enough revenue) to the point where you know you're not getting the profit margin that you want. A great example of what this information allows you to do is hiring a new employee.

Often times we look at employees as their hourly wage and think I can afford $20 per hour. What we forget about is what comes along with an employee; vacation time, uniforms, training time, credentialing (if we are talking about an associate), supplies, computer/workstation etc. Understanding your finances and what each dollar you earn goes to allows you to make more educated decisions. Remember, every dollar that is spent is a dollar that comes off your bottom line (your pocket as the business owner).

The 5 Keys to Understanding Your Practice Financing

Step 1

The first step for understanding practice financing is creating a snapshot of the practice's finances: the long profit-and-loss statements, the balance sheets, the statements of cash flows, etc. Oftentimes, these reports come from a CPA and people don't fully understand these reports; their eyes glaze over when they see them. It can be a lot to look at, which is why you are reading this book though, to find another way to gain an understanding of your practice's finances. When I work with the doctor to change the way that those reports are presented, they have a lightbulb moment, and they really understand the information.

Some doctors want big long profit-and-loss statements. Other doctors like the snapshot version (see next page). For a lot of my clients, I break down the long profit and loss statements or "P&L" and balance sheet (remember not all expenses are on your P&L such as loans or equipment) into expense categories that make sense to an oral surgery practice: personnel, marketing, associate (if applicable), facility, office expenses, owner compensation, equipment, loans, and doctor direct.

Q3 2016 YTD

Category	Amount	% of Product	Industry	% of Income
Production	$ 5,358,431.00			
Income	4,240,485.00			
Collection Rate	79.14%			
Expenses:				
Personnel				
Staff	$ 926,142.57			
	Personnel Total	17.32%		21.89%
Doctor Direct				
	$ 3,514.50			
	Dr. Direct Total	0.07%		0.08%
Marketing				
	$ 16,090.75			
	Marketing Total	0.30%		0.38%
Facility				
	$ 216,048.65			
	Facilities Total	4.03%		5.09%
Supplies				
	$ 387,675.41			
	Dental Supplies Total	7.23%		9.14%
Total Major Expenses	$ 1,551,471.88	28.95%		36.59%
Office Expense (Minor Expenses)				
	$ 120,148.79			
	Minor Expenses Total	2.24%		2.83%
Equipment				
	$ 28,200.63			
	Equipment Total	0.53%		0.67%
Overhead Before Doctor Compensation	$ 1,699,821.30	31.72%		40.09%
Doctor Compensation				
Owners	$ 2,631,732.89			
	Dr. Comp. Total	49.11%		62.06%

We take that big P&L and balance sheet and put it on a one-page snapshot that shows how much they've spent on personnel in their first quarter for example. They can easily say, "I spent X number of dollars on personnel, which was Y percentage of my production, what I billed out, and was Z percentage of the collections which is what actually came in." It is very helpful to understand what your team is costing you each month as personnel is often your largest expense as a business owner.

By doing this month after month, quarter after quarter, year after year, you can watch trends over time garnered from a great amount of information.

When you work with somebody like me, a financial quarterback, we often have benchmark percentages for each of the aforementioned expense categories based on what we've seen from other practices in the industry. You, as the doctor, do not need to know how to create these financial statements. You do, however, need to be able to understand what these statements are telling you about your business. That understanding opens up endless possibilities for taking control of your finances. Something as simple as grouping the expenses into categories and presenting those in a tabular format really makes a big difference.

Step 2

The obvious next step is: What makes up the accounts within each of the categories I mentioned? In terms of personnel, an employee costs more than just their hourly wage. You have to take into account an employee's wages, their payroll tax, benefits such as vacation, holidays, sick days, and continuing education for them.

Surgical assistants, for instance, might need to have continuing education credits for anesthesia certifications, CPR, etc. The cost of uniforms or personal protective equipment also needs to be added into the costs. If all of those things are not taken into consideration then you are underestimating the true cost of employees in your practice. Let's take a look at an example of payroll expense for an employee in MA. Our super assistant Sue earns $20.00/ hr. and works 40 hrs. / week and works all 52 weeks.

There are 2080 working hours in a year, so one may say 2080 x $20 = cost of Sue ($41,600), well, there are taxes you as the employer need to pay on Sue. In reality Sue costs you $45,482.90 or $21.87 per hour. How did I get there? We have MA unemployment (1.87% for new employers applicable for the first $15,000), Federal Unemployment (6% of the first $7,000), FICA (social security (6.2% of first $118,000 and Medicare (1.45% with no earnings limit) for a combines 7.65%. At the start of the year, that is over 15% extra for every hour worked!

For Sue we didn't factor in her two weeks of vacation when you are paying her to not be there her $45,482.90 spread over 2,000 hours rather than 2,080 is 22.74 per hour on average. That's almost $3 per hour, $24 per day, $121 per week that many business owners never think about. Also, don't forget about costs increasing even more if you have to pay your employees for holidays and sick days. More time you are paying for employees when they are not even in the office!

Employees are just one example. We have an entire profit and loss report to review; we cannot just look at the obvious (like hourly wages or monthly rent). If you want to do this, and you understand the breakdown/ snapshot better than the full report, you would just go account by account: Print out your profit-and-loss, and assign each account to an expense category that makes sense to you within your practice. Then look at your balance sheet (compare one from the beginning and end of the period being analyzed) to find changes in equipment, loans, etc.

Once complete, when you see the snapshot, you'll know that personnel includes x, y, and z accounts. You'll know exactly what makes up that category and therefore be able to course correct quickly and appropriately.

There's no cookie-cutter approach to this. Even with subcontractors, we'll dig a little bit deeper. Let's say you don't want to put subcontractors in personnel, for instance. Perhaps you name them as associates or put them in marketing. Maybe you revamped your website this year and had to spend a few thousand dollars for a web developer. You shouldn't count that as personnel; it would go under marketing. Doesn't it make more sense to add this web developer as an expense under marketing than a generic office expense? This snapshot and process is customized for you for the way you want to track expenses and categories. Once you have a template, you'll be able to get consistent valuable data every month, every quarter, and every year, which will really help you moving forward.

Step 3

When you do this, you do need to be careful because benchmarks are great when compared to the correct set of historical data, however, they can be detrimental if you try to compare to anyone that is willing to discuss their practice's finances. This brings us to our third step, using benchmarks. I know it's common for friends to share information and try and get a sanity check on expenses. Be careful with who you are comparing yourself to and be even more careful that you are comparing apples to apples.

My guess is you are not categorizing things in similar manner and that alone will significantly skew results and numbers and will leave you with a potential false comparison, either positive or negative. Let's say you're playing golf with another oral surgeon with whom you went to school. They say, "I only pay 15% of my income on personnel," and you wonder why you're spending 25%. There are so many variables involved, such as how many doctors are in the practice. More doctors mean that you share resources and you share overhead, so that number might go down. Your golf buddy might have a practice in West Virginia, while you're in downtown Boston. Most often, labor will be more expensive downtown in a big city than in the suburbs or in rural West Virginia or rural Maine, for instance. You have to be really careful about who you compare yourself to.

That said there could be two solo practices in the same zip code that have a 10% or a 5% difference in personnel overhead.

It could be that one practice has a practice administrator, which boosts that personnel expense or they may have an extra surgical assistant. An extra annual salary is certainly going to affect your overhead numbers. Long story short, you should be careful what you use for benchmarks and who you compare yourself to. The industry benchmarks are a starting point and the ideal benchmarks are your goals and historical data. I have worked with two clients with very different views on personnel expenses. Both were solo practitioners, however, one has an additional 3 employees. Obviously there is a difference in their percentages paid for staff, however, both practices are healthy financially.

One is on the low end of what we typically to see for a personnel expense and the other is on the higher end, neither is right or wrong, just different.

Step 4

Now that we have our snapshot, from there we can create a budget that works for you, the business owner. Budgeting is a series of choices, it's an art, not a science, and one size does not fit all. Not everybody is going to spend 20% on personnel and 3% on marketing; it's going to fluctuate based upon your situation. As in life, some people want to spend a little bit more on their homes or cars and won't go on as many vacations. Other people would rather go on all kinds of vacations and have smaller houses. It's all about choices.

You have to create goals for yourself. For instance, if you think your personnel expense is a little high, you can aim to bring it down by a few percentage points in a year. How would you do that?

Well you could see more patients to generate more income, or maybe you have excess personnel that got you to where you are but will not bring you where you want to go. What matters is that you're happy with what you have at the end of the day and how you got there. It's your business, they're your finances, and it's your money. People can tell you in which directions they think you should go, but at the end of the day, it's your choice. Your accountant or consultant will try to guide you in certain directions based on their knowledge and experience. When you choose where you want to go, it's their job to help you get there. Remember, in order for them to take you where you want to go, you need to be clear on your goals and vision and communicate these to them.

All of the information that you're going to have allows you to make much better, more informed decisions and to really understand those decisions.

Let's say it's the summer months, and you're extracting a lot of 3rd molars. Your employees have requested summer vacation time off and you could really use another surgical assistant, but you know it's going to cost you $20 an hour to hire them, plus you'll have to pay for retirement, health insurance, and scrubs for them. You'll also have to pay payroll taxes on them. Are you really going to make that money back? If this extra assistant allows you to do even one or two more sets of thirds in a day you will more than make your money back on them. Even if they just turn rooms over, it frees up another assistant to stick with you and do more surgery.

Sometimes, you won't make your money back, but hiring another surgical assistant still makes sense because of the "quality-of-life factor". That plays into the budgeting a bit, sometimes it is worth it to make a little bit less money if you can get home on time for dinner every night. Sometimes that extra time with loved ones is worth more than having a few extra dollars in your pocket.

Just like you have to know exactly how much your employees cost, you need to know how much your office costs (another large expense). Sometimes doctors only think about what they're paying in rent. What about HOA/condo fees? What about utilities? What about when you have to replace the carpet, repaint or pay to get the office cleaned? Doctors tend not to think about this since they're not the big-ticket items.

When you buy a car, you figure out your budget: "I can spend x number of dollars per month;" however, most people don't say, "Well, I also have to pay for car insurance every month, maybe the gas mileage is worse increasing that cost, and this new car will be much more expensive to fix than my last car was." They don't always think of these things as a transportation expenses. Just like you may not think of utilities, landscaping, security, cleaning, etc. as facility expenses for your practice.

Going through finances for your practice is the same way, and these five keys will help you make the decisions and realize what you're spending money on. Are you happy with what you're spending money on? Does it make sense in your industry to be spending in those places?

Step 5

This leads us to our last and "largest" key, what to do with your information. I want to start with a quick story… One of my clients purchased a practice from an owner that didn't keep a close eye on their expenses. During one of my first visits I went into their supply cabinet for a paperclip and found hundreds of pens, packages and packages of white out, sticky notes, pads of paper, calculators. You get the point; it was like they had their own office supply store in house. They would not have to place another order for supplies for years by the looks of it. They had a lot of inventory (most of it useless) because one employee was in charge of ordering, went overboard with it and there was no oversight by the owner. So much money was spent on unnecessary supplies that could become obsolete or simply never be needed.

You don't have to be a penny-pincher, but you own a business. Like Benjamin Franklin said, "A penny saved is a penny earned." If you don't need to spend $5 on a box of paper because you have 3 other boxes, and it takes months to get through 1 box, then don't spend that $5. Unless you're closely looking at your numbers and you understand the information that your accountant, bookkeeper, or consultant is giving you, you really won't realize that you are buying that extra box of paper. You're not going to be aware that the extra box of paper is there or that you don't need that extra box at all. It's not necessarily about the $5.00 ream of paper; this can be extrapolated into anything in your office, gauze, implants, etc.

Another example of waste is related again to personnel. Do you ever have slow afternoons?

Admit it, we all do. Well the next time there is a slow afternoon, and you have a couple of staff members hanging around I want you to consider what it costs you to have everybody there all day (again not just their hourly wage). If they're not busy, it might make sense to let some staff out early that day. You don't need to pay the expense if there's no work being done.

I mentioned that hiring additional staff can come down to quality of life, but if you can't afford it or you realize how much it's going to cost and you're uncomfortable with that, you'd be better off searching for idle capacity within your current staff. Maybe you can move a person from surgery in the morning to the back office in the afternoons to help out in that area with paperwork. Then you don't need to send anybody home, and you don't need to hire another employee. It's a win-win.

We want to create a snapshot based on the way things work in your practice and the way your accountant has your chart of accounts set up. We create these categories, which allow you to have a gauge or a dashboard to understand your financials. You're spending x number of dollars on personnel, x amount on marketing, etc. What makes it more of an art than a science is figuring out what's going to work for you; how much you're comfortable spending on personnel, marketing, and the facility; and how much money you want to take home out of every dollar that comes into the practice as income?

If we work with a Doctor A and a Doctor B, they can figure out what they're each comfortable doing. At the end of the day, if they're both happy, they both feel properly compensated, and they don't feel cash-strapped, then it works. Their budgets could be wildly different from one another, but if it works and they're happy, there's no need to fix something that isn't broken.

You do, however, need to be cognizant of where your money goes. It's easy to lose sight of that in the day-to-day grind. When you're at the office 10 hours a day, seeing patients, doing surgery in-office or at the hospital, doing all of the paperwork, it's exhausting. It's easy to say, "I pay my accountant to look at the numbers. If they're good, I'm good," but you really can't do that. You need to pay attention to what they are saying to you and giving to you so you can get the most value out of them.

If you don't follow one of these five keys, it's not like everything will come crashing down, but they do build on one another, like building blocks.

We create a snapshot, figure out what accounts are in each section, use benchmarks, and make a budget. With that information, you can understand your costs. You can make better decisions. You can combat the peaks and valleys of your industry. You can be in control of your finances.

For instance, if you know how much money you typically make in February versus July in your practice, you can budget and plan for that.

You understand that if your staff expenses are somewhat stagnant through 12 months of the year, but your income has big peaks and valleys, when you're at the peak, you can't take all of the cash out. You have to have some available for the slower times of the year, so you're not cash-strapped.

Some people are financially healthy despite not paying close enough attention to their finances. Plenty of practices have never done this and may not need to. They've always been successful. They have a great staff working under them or an accountant that's really on top of things and extremely involved. Other practices would greatly benefit from going through this process. It's always a good idea, as a business owner, to know where your money is going and how it's working for you.

But, lets think about those successful practices not paying close attention to their finances, not knowing where each dollar goes. Imagine if they did take control of their finances? For example, we were working with a client that was spending $1,200 per month on search engine optimization (SEO) yet their website was not even mobile compatible.

Those $1,200 dollars per month could have gotten them a brand new site that was mobile compatible in 3 months time and then they could take the excess and really look at whether or not they needed to pay all that extra each month to be on the top of Google. This practice has multiple locations (the package they had only allowed their SEO to be focused on one of their locations) yet, the other locations they have still came up at the top of Google when searching Oral surgeon in _____.

They didn't need to pay big money for advertising as they were already well established with a good reputation, and word of mouth was their best referral source.

This one example shows you that you need to pay attention to your overhead. You could be overpaying for something you can have less of, or don't need at all. Remember, as the business owner every dollar saved ends up in your wallet.

If you bring a dollar into the business, how much of that actually ends up in your pocket? Many business owners cannot answer that question. How can you manage your business if you don't understand the financial aspect of it? People don't go into business just for the heck of it. They go into business to make money. They want to make more money working for themselves than they would working for somebody else. To be a doctor, to go through all those years of training, you need to want to help people. You have the mental capacity and the desire to do this, and you're compensated to do this. If you're not paying attention to the compensation side of it, you put yourself behind the eight ball.

Your education, training, facility, and equipment were not free; you also didn't finish your training until ten plus years after many people with a bachelor's degree. This means you have a finite period of time to pay for everything. Yes, in the eye of the public doctors make a lot of money, however, they do not realize the expense incurred to become a surgeon.

An OMS practice can easily cost as much as forty times the average American household income (in September 2014 the US Census Bureau reported median household income to be $51,939). Forty years is a career, that number is someone's lifetime earnings, not something to be taken lightly.

The Common Mistakes Doctors Make with Their Practice Finances

One of the big mistakes doctors make is not taking the time to understand the financial information people are giving to them. You might say, "Oh, Suzy takes care of that for me," but you're embarrassed to ask Suzy what everything means. Not understanding the financial information that people give to you is a big problem. It's accounting and budgeting, and it's not rocket science. You just need to ask the right questions in order to understand.

When you put your full trust in a single person to take care of accounting and budgeting tasks, there's a good chance that that person is ethical, professional, and competent, but putting your full trust in that person and not understanding what they're doing leaves the door open for errors, or worse, embezzlement.

If somebody has full control over your financing, and you pay little attention to the reports that they give you, then you don't know what they're doing on their end. They could be extremely diligent and give you all of the correct information or they could alter the information and be stealing from you without you ever realizing it.

You need to ask questions until you understand what's going on because your livelihood is at stake. You have student loans from years of schooling, and you have to pay for all of your employees, all of the equipment, all of the office supplies, and all of the computers.

The expenses are high. If you don't understand what's happening to the money that comes into the business and how it goes out, you could be leaving an awful lot of money on the table.

The biggest mistake is knowing there's a problem and not taking action. An accountant could say that a doctor is spending way too much money on personnel or their office or that they're taking too much money out of the business in salary. If the doctor doesn't course correct when they know there's a problem, they're going to run into huge financial issues, both personally and professionally. That would be a shame, especially if they had all of the information in front of them the whole time.

Another big mistake is not paying attention to the proper reports. Some doctors' accountants break everything down for them in reports (beyond the financial statements), and they just ignore them because they don't want to deal with them. That could be because of their personality, or they could be burnt out at the end of the day after taking care of patients. Maybe they have young kids at home that they want to see, doctors are people too. Still, putting reports on the back burner isn't something that should happen.

When it comes to your practice's finances, you want to have internal controls in place. It's okay for one person to work on your finances. You're going to have a bookkeeper or an accountant, and at some point, you need to trust them. However, if you don't understand what they're doing and still have full trust in them, that's when you leave the door open for errors that go unnoticed, or worse, as mentioned before, embezzlement.

It only works well if you put full trust in them, they present everything to you—financial reports, bank statements, etc.—and you understand what's going on.

You can get into trouble when you don't have checks and balances in your systems. If someone is reluctant to share information with you, remember that it's your information. It's your business, your bank account, your QuickBooks® account. You should be able to get any information that you want, whenever you want it. The person managing it should be able to show you everything. The conversation should be open and honest.

Doctors need to rely on and trust the information that their CPA gives them while still exercising professional skepticism. You can let them do everything for you and trust them, but make sure you understand what they're saying.

I think a lot of people believe that having a good grasp on this information is much more difficult than it actually is. You don't need to be a CPA or have an accounting degree to understand financial reports. You don't even need to take an accounting class. It's really a matter of the information being presented to you in a way that you understand and that works for you.

You wouldn't sit next to your CPA with an X-ray and expect them to read it correctly Your CPA shouldn't treat you that way either. They should be able to say, "Here's your profit-and-loss statement. Here's your balance sheet. Here's what's going on, and here's why."

Ask questions until you understand. Your CPA, your bookkeeper, and your consultant are all a wealth of knowledge, and they're on your hired team. They want to help you, but you need to help them help you.

Sometimes doctors who have just bought into practices or who are just out of school are not as comfortable with finances as doctors who have owned businesses for 20 years. We started making these snapshots as a way to present information differently to somebody who's not used to looking at financial statements.

I worked with one doctor in particular who had been out of school for a few years. He had been practicing, but he had just purchased his own practice. We were able to work out what expenses we wanted to put into each category and to create goals for our target percentages for the expenses in each category. Now that doctor is well set up to combat the peaks and valleys of the year. He controls his costs; he understands how much his employees cost; and he's able to make educated decisions about whether or not he can add somebody to his team, whether he's spending too much on marketing, whether he's spending too much on staff lunches or referral dinners, etc.

These five keys were developed over a number of years with a variety of different clients. Just like any process, it adapts and evolves. I'll work with a new doctor who asks to see or do something differently, and often they're not the only one who would like to see the information displayed that way. They're not the only one with that question; they were just the one to ask it. This circles back to the idea of making sure you're asking the correct questions.

A lot of doctors focus on their production numbers rather than their income numbers. They charge certain fees, but they're signing contracts with insurances that pay discounted insurance reimbursements. There's an agreed-upon price when those patients come in. That creates an inequality between what they bill out and what they're actually paid on production. You could charge $1,000 to pull a tooth, but if an insurance company will only pay you $200, that $1,000 of production really doesn't mean anything. At the end of the day, you really need to focus on expenses as a function of your income. You can't say, "I pulled 5 teeth today at $1,000 apiece, so I made $5,000 today." If you're only going to get paid $1,000, and you're acting like you made $5,000, then you can't control your costs. You can't control all of the peaks and valleys. You're not really going to care what an employee costs you because you have an inflated number in your mind for what's actually coming into the practice. That can be a sobering realization.

Some doctors may only look at their production numbers because it's easier to get those numbers in real time since they reflect what the doctor actually billed. The only number that matters is what amount of cash actually comes into the practice. You can follow these five keys, but it's not going to work if you're not realistic about what you're looking at. You need to look at revenues and expenses. It's like when you were a kid, and you had a lemonade stand. You thought you would make so much money (well a lot to a child). You made a gallon of lemonade which would be about 16-20 cups at a dollar a cup and you had big dreams of what you would buy with your $20.

But you drank some of it, maybe you weren't great at pouring drinks so you spilled some and if you grew up on a dead end street like me, well there wasn't much traffic, so, you really only got $5 out of it. That's what this is like. You need to pay attention to the $5, not the $20 you wanted to get when you dreamed this up.

How to Understand Your Practice's Finances for a Better Bottom Line

The first step in becoming financially secure is to take a look at all of your financial reports. We'll have a look at your profit-and-loss, your balance sheet, and your statement of cash flows, and have a conversation with you to figure out what's really going on, what makes up all of these different accounts. Everybody portrays insurance expenses differently, for example, so we'll get a good grip on what's going on financially.

Then we'll learn about your practice. How many employees do you have? How long have they been there? What do they do? This will give us a full understanding of what's going on, and then we can start to create a snapshot and figure out what percentage goes in each bucket. We'll determine whether you're happy with that and whether it's in line with industry standards.

Maybe you want to take more money home at the end of the day, or you feel like you're spending too much money on personnel. Maybe something doesn't feel right, but you don't know what it is. Creating a snapshot and figuring out which accounts go into each category of the snapshot will help you budget and create goals. If something is not right financially in your business, it's not going to be fixed overnight. The snapshot makes it easier for you to see when categories fluctuate so that you can make adjustments and corrections.

Once we get that initial plan in place, we're going to look for sustainable progress towards your goal, month after month, quarter after quarter, and year after year. We want to be able to combat the peaks and valleys every year, to be prepared for those moments, or to be prepared for the big expenses that come once a year. Let's say you have a $10,000 insurance premium due in January every year. You could either take that $10,000 hit in January, or, if you plan for it, you could space $10,000 evenly over 12 months putting a little aside each month. That would be much less of a hit. Things like that do wonders for cash flow.

Another big hurdle that you may have during this process of creating budgets and goals is simply not wanting to change things because it's the way they've always been done. In one practice I worked with the owner started paying a bonus in December and a bonus in the summer just because it had always been done that way. The bonus was not tied to anything other than the employees just showing up. This had been going on for about 20 years. Can you imagine how much extra this practice was paying in personnel expenses without even realizing it? Their personnel expenses had gotten out of control but they couldn't figure out why. As you can imagine paying two bonuses per year adds up very quickly, especially if the bonus is equivalent to a paycheck. Your personnel expense will quickly get out of hand doing this.

If you spend 35% on personnel and are looking to lower that number (that is high and should be reduced by a good amount), and you give two sizeable bonuses each year, maybe you need to cut back on the bonuses.

Bonuses are supposed to be rewards. They're supposed to be rewarded when the company does really well, and you want to thank the staff. Paying staff two bonuses every year is no different than paying everybody a few extra dollars an hour at the end of the day. You need to strive to be efficient while also keeping your employees happy. I am not saying you should be Ebenezer Scrooge here and be a penny pincher, however, you do not need to give large bonuses because that is what was always done.

Also, you need to know that you can't change things overnight, but you can change your habits and reduce your expenses in some area. You can shift where you're spending money. If you're comfortable with your income and would rather have a nicer office than an extra staff member, that's something you can play with. Again, there's no cookie-cutter approach. It's really a matter of getting the information and gaining an understanding of your practice, your goals, and the way things work for you. Then we can create an agreed-upon approach together.

For example, some surgeons have children in high school. They are going to need extra cash to pay for their children's college educations. That becomes a priority over getting new chairs, or new computers, even hiring an extra staff member. Or, lets say you just purchased an office that is out of date and you don't have any large financial commitments in the near future, you may be more apt to put every extra dollar back into the business to make it more welcoming, more efficient, or even bring it into the EMR era from paper charts.

The point is, everyone is different, as is their business, so, if you know yourself and you know your business, there's nothing stopping you from taking control of your finances and having your plan put into action.

If you have questions, go to our website: **terribradleyconsulting.com**. You can also email me at ben@terribradleyconsulting.com, or you can call us at 844-762-4667. I would be happy to talk to you about what's going on or answer any questions you have.

The 5 Keys to Confidence and Understanding Your Practice Financing…

You went through years of training to become a top oral surgeon, but probably were never properly taught how to evaluate financial reports. You would never expect an accountant to evaluate a radiograph, so why is it assumed you should be able to read and comprehend complex financial statements from your CPA?

That's where we come in. We help oral surgeons just like you understand your OMS practice finances so you can manage your practice to be more efficient, all the while reducing your stress and improving your bottom line.

Step 1: Perform an in depth analysis and discovery to help us better understand your unique situation and create an easy to understand financial snapshot of where your practice is now.

Step 2: Decide what accounts will make up each section of the snapshot.

Step 3: Use benchmarks. Remember that not all industries or business within the same industry are the same.

Step 4: Budget. Create a plan that makes sense for you.

Step 5: You now have this valuable information, what do you do with it? You start to make more informed decisions about your practice and get a grip on your practice finances.

As an oral surgeon, spending the majority of your time in the clinical side is where you should be. As a business owner, the better you understand the financial side of your practice the more profitable you can be.

Now you can build confidence in and heighten your understanding of your OMS practice finances so you can achieve your practice goals. We are here to help; send an email to me at: **Ben@TerriBradleyconsulting.com** I would be happy to talk to you about anything mentioned in this short book, or anything we did not cover.

www.ingramcontent.com/pod-product-compliance
Lightning Source LLC
Chambersburg PA
CBHW071436200326
41520CB00014B/3711